A CONCISE SUMMARY OF **DR. WILLIAM DAVIS'S**

Wheat Belly

...in 30 minutes

A 30 MINUTE HEALTH SUMMARY

GARAMOND
PRESS

TABLE OF CONTENTS

Introduction   2

Chapter Summaries

Chapter 1: *What* Belly?   4

Chapter 2: Not Your Grandma's Muffins: The Creation of Modern Wheat   7

Chapter 3: Wheat Deconstructed   10

Chapter 4: Hey, Man, Wanna Buy Some Exorphins? The Addictive Properties of Wheat   13

Chapter 5: Your Wheat Belly Is Showing: The Wheat/Obesity Connection   16

Chapter 6: Hello, Intestine. It's Me, Wheat. Wheat and Celiac Disease   19

Chapter 7: Diabetes Nation: Wheat and Insulin Resistance   22

Chapter 8: Dropping Acid: Wheat as the Great pH Disrupter   25

Chapter 9: Cataracts, Wrinkles, and Dowager's Humps: Wheat and the Aging Process   28

Chapter 10: My Particles Are Bigger Than Yours: Wheat and Heart Disease   31

Chapter 11: It's All in Your Head: Wheat and the Brain   34

Chapter 12: Bagel Face: Wheat's Destructive Effect on the Skin   37

Chapter 13: Goodbye, Wheat: Create a Healthy, Delicious, Wheat-Free Life   40

Conclusion   43

INTRODUCTION

Overview

In *Wheat Belly*, Dr. William Davis makes the case that eliminating wheat will lead to a healthier life. Through personal experiences, clinical studies, and an exploration of the diseases and medical conditions associated with different diets, Davis details the damaging effects that modern, genetically manipulated wheat has had on the human body.

Since it was first introduced as einkorn wheat in its most ancient form, wheat has been genetically manipulated to create faster-yielding, higher-performing, better-tasting versions of itself. Davis suggests that through this process, wheat has also become incompatible with human digestion. Ironically, due to a shift in nutritional guidelines in the past fifty years, people are consuming wheat in unprecedented amounts, believing that whole grains are essential to a balanced diet. The results are dramatic. Davis explores wheat's adverse effects on the entire body, from the blood to the heart to the visceral organs to the skin, presenting a wheat-free diet as the ultimate solution. He promises that once wheat is eliminated, weight loss, better sleep, and overall better health will follow.

About the Author

William Davis, MD, is a cardiologist who uses a wheat-free approach not only to prevent but also to reverse heart disease in his patients. He is medical director and creator of the Track Your Plaque program, a program that outlines how to use CT heart scans to detect, track, and control coronary plaque. His previous book, *Track Your Plaque*, describes this program in detail. Davis is a consultant for the nutritional supplement industry and serves as vice president for cardiology for Obesity PPM, a consulting firm that offers solutions to the obesity crisis. He has been published in the *American Journal of Therapeutics* and *Life Extension Magazine*, and contributes frequently to health websites.

How the Book Came About

Dr. Davis first came to question the idea of a healthy diet high in whole grains when he noticed a photo of himself from a family vacation in Florida. While he jogged five miles a day and ate a sensible, balanced diet, in the photo he was clearly fat, at least thirty pounds overweight. When he made this discovery, Davis was in the midst of devising a unique strategy for helping his diabetic and prediabetic patients lose weight, one that lowered glucose (blood sugar) levels by eliminating wheat. Many of the patients dropped thirty to forty pounds, and they also reported improved energy, deeper sleep, and the disappearance of a variety of symptoms, ranging from abdominal cramping to rashes to asthma. Davis was intrigued. What began as a weight-loss strategy turned into a deeper exploration of wheat and its effects, mostly damaging, on the human body. In the *New York Times* best seller *Wheat Belly*, Davis describes what he uncovered.

1

WHAT BELLY?

Overview

Mainstream dietary recommendations over the past few decades are to eat less fat and sugar and more whole grains. Yet Americans have increasingly become obese. Davis says this is because we consume foods that contain wheat products at nearly every meal. Studies show that wheat, which has a higher glycemic index (the measure of how much a particular food increases the blood sugar level) than refined sugar, is a direct cause of abdominal weight gain. *Wheat Belly* proposes that by eliminating wheat from their diet, people can reduce belly fat and become thinner, healthier, and more energetic. Signs of diabetes and inflammatory diseases such as arthritis and asthma may also be reduced or eliminated.

> *"Advice to cut fat and cholesterol intake and replace the calories with whole grains that was issued by the National Heart, Lung, and Blood Institute through its National Cholesterol Education Program in 1985 coincides precisely with the start of a sharp upward climb in body weight for men and women."*
>
> — Dr. William Davis, *Wheat Belly*

Chapter Summary

As dietary recommendations have created a national trend to cut back on fats and sugars and replace these with whole grains, there has been a marked increase in waistlines and a noticeable decline in overall health—even among people who exercise regularly. According to Davis, wheat has come to dominate Americans' diets, making people fat and unhealthy.

Whole wheat bread, with a glycemic index of 72, raises blood sugar levels more than sugar, with a glycemic index of 59. When blood sugar levels rise, more insulin is produced. Insulin is a hormone that, among other functions, tells the body to store fat.

Fat stored in the central part of the body, known as visceral fat, provokes inflammatory responses in the body (which can lead to diseases such as arthritis), disrupts the insulin response (which can lead to diabetes), and sends abnormal metabolic signals to the rest of the body (which can lead to overeating). This visceral fat, sometimes called a beer belly, Davis calls "wheat belly" because it represents the accumulation of fat that results from years of consuming wheat-related products.

According to Davis, the simple cure for wheat belly and its accompanying ailments is to eliminate wheat from the diet. Once wheat is gone, he says excess weight will melt away, energy and focus will improve, and even diseases such as diabetes may be lessened or cured.

"[F]or the most bang for your buck, eliminating wheat is the easiest and most effective step you can take to safeguard your health and trim your waistline."

— Dr. William Davis, *Wheat Belly*

Chapter 1: Key Points

- The dramatic increase in consumption of whole grains over the past few decades has paralleled a similar surge in obesity and diabetes rates.

- Wheat has a high glycemic index and is the largest source of gluten in the human diet; studies show that these components can be directly linked to abdominal weight gain and an increased risk of diabetes.

- A wheat-free diet has the potential to promote weight loss and improve health.

2

NOT YOUR GRANDMA'S MUFFINS: THE CREATION OF MODERN WHEAT

Overview

From bread to breakfast cereal to pasta, wheat accounts for 20 percent of all calories consumed on earth. But wheat has been genetically altered to such a degree that modern wheat bears very little resemblance to the original einkorn wheat our ancestors ate ten thousand years ago. While these alterations have increased yield and decreased production costs, they have also created modern strains of wheat that may be difficult for humans to digest and harmful to our health.

"Modern wheat, despite all the genetic alterations to modify hundreds, if not thousands, of its genetically determined characteristics, made its way to the worldwide human food supply with nary a question surrounding its suitability for human consumption."

— Dr. William Davis, *Wheat Belly*

Chapter Summary

Wheat was first harvested by the Natufians around 8500 b.c. to supplement their hunter-gatherer diet. This ancestor of modern wheat, einkorn, was much different genetically than its modern equivalent; most notably it had a simple genetic code with only fourteen chromosomes. Einkorn crossed with a wild grass yielded emmer, the wheat that was around in biblical times. Emmer was eventually crossed with another natural grass, yielding *Triticum aestivum*—a complex wheat containing forty-two chromosomes that was genetically easy to manipulate.

Fifty years ago, intense manipulation began. Modern wheat is descended from strains created at the International Maize and Wheat Improvement Center, an agricultural research program developed to increase the yield of soy, corn, and wheat, and thus reduce world hunger. Founded in 1943, this program hybridized, or crossbred, existing strains of wheat. By 1980, it had created thousands of strains of wheat that, thanks to human intervention, were hundreds of genes apart from the original einkorn wheat.

No safety testing was ever done on these hybrid crops. It was simply assumed that since the wheat was still a form of wheat, it would be safe. But analysis of the proteins in modern hybrid wheat found that while about 95 percent of the proteins expressed in the offspring are present in both the parent strains, 5 percent are unique and are found in neither parent. So what we know about the safety of the parent strains may or may not be true of the hybrid strains.

In addition, modern wheat *(Triticum aestivum)* expresses a higher number of genes that make gluten proteins. Gluten makes bread more stretchy and pliable, and makes it rise more. But it comes at the cost of causing greater blood sugar spikes.

*"Small changes in wheat protein structure can spell
the difference between a devastating immune response
to wheat protein versus no immune response at all."*

— Dr. William Davis, *Wheat Belly*

Chapter 2: Key Points

- Modern wheat has been altered dramatically since the first hybridization efforts in 1943. It is the result of direct genetic manipulation by humans over the past fifty years.

- Despite extensive genetic alterations, hybridized wheat has not been tested to determine its safety for humans or animals.

- Modern wheat contains more gluten—a protein that causes spikes in blood sugar.

3

WHEAT DECONSTRUCTED

Overview

What kinds of carbohydrates you eat are even more important than how many. Carbohydrates that are more easily and rapidly digested create spikes in blood sugar, causing the body to make more insulin. The spikes are followed by crashes that leave us hungry. Wheat is high in a type of carbohydrate that is very efficiently digested, causing it to have the same effect on the body as candy or sugary soda drinks. The repeated spikes in blood sugar and increased insulin production promote fat storage and can lead to diabetes. Davis suggests that following a wheat-free diet will lead to lower blood sugar levels and less incidence of obesity and diabetes.

"[W]heat products elevate blood sugar levels more than virtually any other carbohydrate, from beans to candy bars. This has important implications for body weight, since glucose is unavoidably accompanied by insulin, the hormone that allows entry of glucose into the cells of the body, converting the glucose to fat."

— Dr. William Davis, *Wheat Belly*

Chapter Summary

Wheat is a complex carbohydrate, meaning it is composed of repeating chains of glucose (simple carbohydrates like processed sugar are made of just one or two chains of glucose). Conventional wisdom says complex carbs are better for you because they break down more slowly in the digestive tract.

But modern *Triticum aestivum* wheat contains a very easily digestible form of these complex carbs called amylopectin A. These carbs are more efficiently converted to blood sugar than most other carbs, simple or complex. So when you look at how quickly and efficiently whole wheat bread breaks down into glucose, it's about the same in your body as a can of soda. You just get more fiber from the whole wheat.

Amylopectin A, because it is digested so efficiently and quickly, induces a blood glucose peak that lasts about two hours, followed by a crash as glucose levels drop. Insulin levels increase as glucose levels rise, because insulin is required to metabolize glucose. This glucose-insulin cycle acts as an appetite stimulant, and also causes the body to store more visceral fat. Stored visceral fat causes a poorer response to insulin, causing the body to require higher and higher levels of insulin—a situation that sets you up for diabetes.

The other problem with wheat is gluten. Glutens are the storage proteins in wheat, and are what make it stretchy and easy to rise. Hybridized wheat has been engineered to increase the types of glutens that make wheat good for baking. But these types of glutens also tend to provoke inflammatory and allergic responses in the body.

"The bigger your wheat belly, the poorer your response to insulin, since the deep visceral fat of the wheat belly is associated with poor responsiveness, or 'resistance,' to insulin, demanding higher and higher insulin levels, a situation that cultivates diabetes."

— Dr. William Davis, *Wheat Belly*

Chapter 3: Key Points

- The way the body processes the carbohydrates in wheat can result in increased abdominal fat and overall health issues.

- The amylopectin A carbohydrates in wheat cause blood sugar levels to spike, leading to elevated insulin levels and visceral fat storage. Studies show that eliminating these carbohydrates from the diet should lead to weight loss.

- The gluten proteins present in modern wheat, while making wheat better for baking, can also trigger inflammatory reactions.

4

HEY, MAN, WANNA BUY SOME EXORPHINS? THE ADDICTIVE PROPERTIES OF WHEAT

Overview

According to Davis, wheat is one of the few foods that can change our behavior and alter our moods. Studies show that when people completely eliminate wheat from their diets, they initially experience feelings of withdrawal; only eating wheat can alleviate these feelings. Additional studies observe that people suffering from schizophrenia, autism, and ADHD experience more severe symptoms of the diseases when wheat is present in their diets. These findings suggest that adopting a wheat-free diet will potentially improve mood and overall health.

"[W]heat is one of the few foods that can alter behavior, induce pleasurable effects, and generate a withdrawal syndrome upon its removal."

— Dr. William Davis, *Wheat Belly*

Chapter Summary

According to Davis, wheat induces feelings of pleasure for some people. When interpreted as cravings, these feelings can eventually lead to a wheat addiction. As wheat is digested, the glutens degrade to a mix of special polypeptides (chains of amino acids that form part of a protein molecule) that are able to penetrate the blood-brain barrier that separates the brain from the bloodstream. Once these special polypeptides, called exorphins, enter the brain, they bind to the brain's morphine receptors. Scientists believe these exorphins are responsible for a wheat-induced feeling of euphoria and the associated addictive response. In experiments, when the exorphins are blocked, people eat less wheat and lose weight.

Dr. F. Curtis Dohan at the Veterans Administration Hospital in Philadelphia observed that exorphins also affect the moods and behaviors of patients suffering from schizophrenia. After four weeks on a wheat-free diet, doctors reported the patients experienced reduced auditory hallucinations, fewer delusions, and less detachment from reality. When they placed these same patients back on a diet that included wheat, the symptoms resumed normal levels. Studies suggest that autistic children and those suffering from ADHD may also show improved behavior on a gluten-free diet, although these findings are less conclusive. While Davis says it is unlikely wheat *caused* these problems, it appears to be associated with worsening of the symptoms.

Davis claims that wheat is one of very few foods shown to alter moods and create addictive behaviors. Taking it one step further, he suggests that because wheat can cause pleasure, pushing us to want more, it is an appetite stimulant. Continuing this argument, Davis says a wheat-free diet will diminish hunger and cravings, and lead to fewer mood swings, improved ability to concentrate, and deeper sleep.

"Understanding that wheat, specifically exorphins from gluten, have the potential to generate euphoria, addictive behavior, and appetite stimulation means that we have a potential means of weight control: Lose the wheat, lose the weight."

— Dr. William Davis, *Wheat Belly*

Chapter 4: Key Points

- When wheat is digested, gluten is degraded to a mix of exorphins that can bind to the brain's morphine receptors, creating feelings of euphoria and driving a desire to consume more wheat, creating an addiction.

- Eliminating wheat from the diet breaks the addiction and will diminish hunger and lead to a better mood, improved ability to concentrate, and deeper sleep.

- Doctors have observed that consumption of wheat worsens the symptoms of schizophrenia, autism, and ADHD.

5

YOUR WHEAT BELLY IS SHOWING: THE WHEAT/OBESITY CONNECTION

Overview

According to Davis, the dramatic rise of obesity and diabetes in the United States came at the same time that nutritional experts began advising us to eat more whole grains. In an effort to be healthy, Americans began eating wheat in unprecedented amounts, driving blood sugar levels higher. These spikes in blood sugar led to an accompanying growth of visceral fat, a dangerous type of fat that surrounds the organs and has been linked to diabetes, dementia, heart disease, and colon cancer. Davis suggests that removing wheat from the diet promotes weight loss because it eliminates spikes in blood sugar and its accompanying visceral fat gain.

"I'd like to make the case that foods made with or containing wheat make you fat. I'd go as far as saying that overly enthusiastic wheat consumption is the main cause of the obesity and diabetes crisis in the United States."

— Dr. William Davis, *Wheat Belly*

Chapter Summary

Recommendations to consume more whole grains are primarily based on two findings. The first is real evidence that when processed grain flour products are replaced with whole grain flour products, there is a reduction of colon cancer, heart disease, and diabetes. The second is observations that suggest higher dietary fat intake is associated with higher cholesterol levels and risk for heart disease. But increasing wheat consumption, even whole grains, has never been proven to be a healthy diet.

Wheat triggers a cycle of insulin-driven satiety and hunger that lead to the deposition of visceral fat. This fat accumulates around the liver, kidneys, pancreas, abdomen, and intestines. Visceral fat is unique in its ability to trigger the body's inflammatory responses. The specific response triggered by visceral fat underlies diabetes, hypertension, heart disease, dementia, arthritis, and colon cancer.

Visceral fat also produces estrogen in both men and women. Increased visceral fat has been associated with an increased risk for breast cancer in women. It stimulates the growth of breast tissue in men, leading to "man boobs."

People with celiac disease have an inflammatory response to gluten that destroys the lining of their intestines. Remove all gluten, and the lining regenerates and health is restored. Experts on the disease have observed that increasingly, newly diagnosed patients are overweight or obese. Studies show that simply removing all gluten products from their diet, with no other intervention, causes dramatic weight loss.

While commercial gluten-free foods do not trigger the inflammatory responses that characterize celiac disease, they usually replace gluten with starches. These starches still trigger the glucose-insulin responses that cause weight gain. So a healthy diet completely eliminates all sources of amylopectin A, and that includes starches.

"Wheat elimination is a vastly underappreciated strategy for rapid and profound weight loss, particularly from visceral fat."

— Dr. William Davis, *Wheat Belly*

Chapter 5: Key Points

- The wheat belly phenomenon explains why people who follow otherwise healthy lifestyles still end up being overweight.

- Wheat consumption leads to an increase in visceral fat. Visceral fat triggers inflammatory responses that can lead to serious diseases. It also produces estrogen in both men and women.

- Studies show that simply removing wheat products from the diet can lead to dramatic weight loss.

6

HELLO, INTESTINE. IT'S ME, WHEAT. WHEAT AND CELIAC DISEASE

Overview

The most dramatic manifestation of wheat intolerance is celiac disease, and its diagnosis has increased fourfold in the past fifty years. According to Davis, this surge in celiac incidence is a result of the modern genetic modifications made to wheat and, in particular, gluten proteins. Celiac disease breaks down the lining of the small intestine, allowing antibodies and bacteria into the bloodstream and causing abnormal inflammatory and immune responses. Its mechanism may be responsible for a wide range of diseases that all relate back to gluten intolerance.

"[T]he increase in celiac disease has been paralleled by an increase in type 1 diabetes, autoimmune diseases such as multiple sclerosis and Crohn's disease, and allergies."

— Dr. William Davis, *Wheat Belly*

Chapter Summary

Research suggests that the incidence of celiac disease has increased fourfold over the past fifty years. The rise in the number of effected people can be partially attributed to better diagnostics, but researchers agree that the true incidence is also on the rise. They do not agree about why, though. This increase has been paralleled by an increase in type 1 diabetes and in autoimmune diseases such as multiple sclerosis, Crohn's disease, and allergies.

Wheat may be part of the explanation. Researchers in the Netherlands compared modern strains of wheat with strains that were widely available until a century ago, and found that celiac-triggering gluten proteins were expressed in higher levels in modern wheat, while non-celiac-triggering proteins were expressed less.

When people who suffer from celiac disease eat anything that contains gluten, the gliadin protein of gluten breaks down the lining of their small intestines, making it permeable. As the lining gets damaged, it allows the various products of digestion, as well as helpful bacteria from the small intestine, to enter the bloodstream. When substances that are not supposed to escape from the intestines do, one effect is autoimmunity—the immune system believes the body is under attack and attacks itself.

Although diarrhea and abdominal cramping are the most common signs of celiac disease, in many cases the signs are atypical, such as anemia, skin rash, allergies, or migraine headaches, or there are no immediate signs of disease. The problem then goes undiagnosed.

While celiac is a damaging disease on its own, it is made even more dangerous by the accompanying conditions prevalent in celiac sufferers, including rashes, liver disease, autoimmune diseases, insulin-dependent diabetes, neurological impairments, and nutritional deficiencies. Davis proposes that this represents a wider (beyond celiac disease) immune-mediated gluten intolerance. In addition, he says irritable bowel syndrome and acid reflux disease may represent what he calls "lesser forms of celiac disease."

"[T]he reach of gluten consumption consequences is mind-bogglingly wide. It can affect any organ at any age. . . . Thinking of celiac disease as just diarrhea, as is often the case in many doctors' offices, is an enormous, and potentially fatal, oversimplification."

— Dr. William Davis, *Wheat Belly*

Chapter 6: Key Points

- People who cannot tolerate gluten proteins suffer from celiac disease.

- Celiac disease causes abnormal inflammatory and immune responses because it deteriorates the lining of the small intestine, allowing the products of digestion and bacteria from the small intestine to enter the bloodstream.

- The increased incidence of celiac disease is paralleled by an increase in the incidences of type 1 diabetes, various autoimmune diseases, and allergies. This may be indicative of a wider immune-mediated gluten intolerance.

DIABETES NATION:
WHEAT AND INSULIN RESISTANCE

Overview

A sharp increase in the incidence of diabetes in the United States since the 1980s coincides with a shift to a diet low in fats and proteins and high in grain products. Wheat causes blood sugar levels to spike, triggering the release of insulin and an accompanying growth of visceral fat. After years of this repetitive process, diabetes develops. Davis argues that nutrition, not medication, is the best treatment for diabetes. Research shows that greatly lowering carbohydrate intake can improve or reverse diabetes in many patients.

> *"In short, remove wheat and thereby reverse a* constellation *of phenomena that would otherwise result in diabetes and all its associated health consequences, three or four medications if not seven, and years shaved off your life."*
> — Dr. William Davis, *Wheat Belly*

Chapter Summary

The number of Americans with type 2 diabetes is growing faster than the number of Americans with any other disease condition except obesity. An additional 22 to 39 percent of American adults have prediabetes (higher than normal blood glucose levels). At the same time, per capita consumption of wheat products has increased by twenty-six pounds a year since 1970. The average American across all age brackets now eats 133 pounds of wheat a year.

Davis believes this is not a coincidence. As the body accumulates visceral fat, insulin resistance develops and the number of beta cells in the pancreas (cells responsible for producing insulin) increases by as much as 50 percent to meet the body's growing need for insulin. But very high blood sugar levels also cause glucotoxicity, where the beta cells are damaged by high blood sugar. Beta cells are also damaged by lipotoxicity, which results from increased triglycerides and fatty acids—levels of which also rise after repeated carbohydrate ingestion. Pancreatic damage is further worsened by inflammatory phenomena caused by visceral fat. Over time, enough beta cells are damaged for type 2 diabetes to develop.

Davis says eliminating wheat from your diet is the single most effective thing you can do to lower your risk of developing diabetes, because you then escape the glucose-insulin cycle of appetite and blood sugar spikes. When appetite is reduced, caloric intake is reduced, visceral fat disappears, insulin resistance improves, and blood sugar levels fall.

The American Diabetes Association diet recommends 135 to 180 grams of "healthy whole grains" a day, combined with low fat intake, but Davis asserts that eating carbohydrates can make the damage to the pancreas only worse. Research has demonstrated that a sharp reduction in dietary carbohydrates reverses insulin resistance, distortions in blood sugar after eating, and visceral fat.

> *"The concept that diabetes should be regarded as a disease of carbohydrate intolerance is beginning to gain ground in the medical community."*
> — Dr. William Davis, *Wheat Belly*

In type 1 diabetes, which typically develops in children, antibodies to insulin and beta cells result in autoimmune destruction of the pancreas. The incidence of type 1 diabetes is also increasing. This coincides with an increase in the incidence of celiac disease—and with the appearance of genetically modified wheat. Children with celiac disease are ten times more likely to develop type 1 diabetes. Davis says research is needed into whether eliminating wheat at birth can avert the development of type 1 diabetes, especially in children with a genetic predisposition.

Chapter 7: Key Points

- The dramatic increase in diabetes since the mid-1980s has been paralleled by a dramatic increase in obesity; wheat consumption and its accompanying blood sugar surges contribute greatly to this rise in both obesity and diabetes.

- The detrimental effects of visceral fat on the body are linked to the mechanisms that cause diabetes.

- Diabetes can be controlled, and even cured, by adopting a diet that strictly limits carbohydrate consumption and naturally reduces blood sugar levels.

DROPPING ACID:
WHEAT AS THE GREAT PH DISRUPTER

Overview

According to Davis, altering the body's healthy pH level of 7.4 by just 0.5 in either the acidic or alkaline direction is dangerous. Wheat products, which release high levels of sulfuric acid, effectively tip the balance to the acidic side. When the body senses an overabundance of acid, it draws calcium (an alkali) from the bones, which can leave them dangerously depleted. Wheat can also cause the cartilage that cushions the joints to become stiff and brittle. Davis suggests that removing wheat from the diet can alleviate these conditions.

"[W]heat exerts direct and indirect bone- and joint-destructive effects in any wheat-consuming human."

— Dr. William Davis, *Wheat Belly*

Chapter Summary

For the body to function properly, it needs to maintain a pH of 7.4. Foods that come from animal sources, such as meats and cheeses, are acidic—although animal proteins also exert a bone-strengthening effect by triggering the production of a hormone called IGF-1, which spurs bone growth and mineralization. Eating vegetables and fruits, which are alkaline, can also counterbalance the acidic effects of meats. Grains are the only plant products that generate acids. Wheat is particularly acidic, yielding more sulfuric acid per gram than any meat. A typical Western diet, dominated by meat and wheat products, tips the body's pH toward the acidic.

An acidic pH triggers the body to draw calcium (an alkali) from the bones and stimulates cells within the bones to dissolve bone tissue in an effort to release their calcium more quickly. Davis suggests that both of these processes deplete the bones of calcium, causing them to become brittle and frail.

Davis says wheat also plays a role in arthritis. Arthritis, long thought to be a complication of the wear and tear of excess weight on the joints, is an inflammation process, and Davis reminds us that excess visceral fat causes inflammation. Studies show that losing visceral fat improves arthritis more than can be expected from weight loss alone.

Glycation is another process that can complicate arthritis. Glycation is a reaction that takes place when simple sugar molecules become attached to proteins or fats. This results in the formation of rogue molecules known as advanced glycation end products (AGEs), which cause protein fibers to become stiff and malformed. Cartilage, which cushions the joints, is especially susceptible to glycation because cartilage cells do not reproduce; once they are damaged, they remain damaged. Consuming wheat increases blood glucose levels and causes glycation. Since damage due to glycation is cumulative, the more wheat ingested, the more harmful the effects.

*"Modern eating patterns therefore create
a chronic acidosis that in turn leads us to
osteoporosis, bone fragility, and fractures."*
— Dr. William Davis, *Wheat Belly*

Chapter 8: Key Points

- Although the human body strives to maintain a healthy pH of 7.4, the consumption of wheat, which is acidic, challenges this balance.

- When the body's pH is too acidic, it is forced to pull calcium carbonate and calcium phosphate from bones. This leaves them brittle and frail.

- Glycation causes joint stiffness and can cause cartilage to become brittle, leading to arthritis. Sustained consumption of wheat can lead to joint inflammation, pain, and arthritis.

9

CATARACTS, WRINKLES, AND DOWAGER'S HUMPS: WHEAT AND THE AGING PROCESS

Overview

AGEs are molecules that form when glucose binds to protein. These molecules accumulate in the body's organs, where they interfere with normal functioning, triggering the effects of aging. Davis suggests that consuming large quantities of wheat accelerates this process by supplying the blood with high levels of sustained glucose that can be converted to AGEs. He hypothesizes that a diet low in wheat should have the opposite effect, slowing the parts of the aging process affected by AGEs.

> *"Wheat, because of its unique blood glucose-increasing effect, makes you age faster. Via its blood sugar/AGE-increasing effects, wheat accelerates the rate at which you develop signs of skin aging, kidney dysfunction, dementia, atherosclerosis, and arthritis."*
>
> — Dr. William Davis, *Wheat Belly*

Chapter Summary

Advanced glycation end products, or AGEs (introduced in the previous chapter), are essentially useless debris that accumulates in the organs and results in tissue decay. They can cause stiffened arteries, cataracts, dementia, loss of skin tone, and other deteriorations that signal the aging process. The stiffening caused by AGEs is irreversible, and the older people get, the more AGEs can be found in all their organs.

AGEs are found in some foods, but are also a byproduct of high blood sugar. In people with extremely high blood sugar levels, such as diabetics, AGEs can accelerate the aging process. The higher the blood sugar and the longer blood sugars stay elevated, the more AGEs accumulate, creating a faster buildup and a more noticeable impact. Many diabetics in their twenties and thirties suffer from atherosclerosis, kidney disease, and neuropathy—diseases most commonly found in people ages sixty and over. AGEs are also responsible for most of the complications of diabetes.

AGEs also form when blood sugar is normal—although at a much lower rate. But consuming large quantities of wheat products, because of their effects on blood sugar, can cause AGEs to form and accelerate the changes associated with aging.

HbA1c is a blood test that gauges the rate of AGE formation by measuring the average plasma glucose concentration over prolonged periods of time; the higher the average blood glucose levels, the higher the HbA1c. According to Davis, the higher a body's HbA1c level, the faster it is aging, as well. When foods that increase blood glucose levels, such as wheat, are ingested regularly, they tend to increase HbA1c levels. Davis proposes that a diet low in wheat should, therefore, slow the aging process, although this has not yet been studied.

*"[F]oods that increase blood glucose levels the most
and are consumed more frequently are reflected
by higher levels of HbA1c that in turn reflect a
faster rate of organ damage and aging."*

— Dr. William Davis, *Wheat Belly*

Chapter 9: Key Points

- AGEs are protein-glucose molecules that contribute to the effects of aging, including stiffened arteries, cataracts, loss of skin tone, and interrupted neurological connections in the brain.

- The higher the blood sugar and the longer blood sugars stay elevated, the more AGEs accumulate.

- The higher the body's AGE level, the faster it is aging; foods that increase blood glucose, such as wheat, cause higher levels of AGEs.

MY PARTICLES ARE BIGGER THAN YOURS: WHEAT AND HEART DISEASE

Overview

Diets high in carbohydrates stimulate the production of insulin, which triggers fatty acid synthesis in the liver. The liver releases these fatty acids in the form of triglycerides—which provide energy for metabolic processes. Through the processes of metabolism, triglycerides are turned into small particles called low-density lipoproteins (LDLs)—particles that carry fatty acids through the bloodstream. The more insulin, the more triglycerides, and the more triglycerides, the smaller the LDLs. These very small LDLs linger in the body and can build up in the lining walls of the arteries and lead to heart disease and stroke.

"Anything that provokes an increase in blood sugar will also, in parallel, provoke small LDL particles. Anything that keeps blood sugar from increasing, such as proteins, fats, and reduction in carbohydrates such as wheat, reduces small LDL particles."

— Dr. William Davis, *Wheat Belly*

Chapter Summary

Davis says LDL particles are not cholesterol, although they are typically thought of that way in the medical and pharmaceutical communities. The precursor of these LDL particles are very-low-density lipoprotein particles (VLDLs), which are produced in the liver. VLDLs are a package of proteins and fatty acids in the form of triglycerides and cholesterol. In the bloodstream, they transport these fatty acids to peripheral tissues and metabolize them to be absorbed. What is left behind are LDL particles, which are eventually taken up by the liver.

The size of the LDL particles depends on how much triglyceride the VLDLs give up. The more they give up, the smaller the resulting LDL particle.

While large LDL particles are easily recognized by receptor cells in the liver and taken up for disposal, small LDL particles are less easily recognized and remain in the bloodstream longer. They are more likely to be taken up by inflammatory white cells that reside in the walls of arteries and form atherosclerotic plaque—a deposit of fat that accumulates in the lining of the arteries. Numerous studies show that the presence of atherosclerotic plaque increases the likelihood of having a heart attack or stroke.

While carbohydrates contain almost no triglycerides themselves, they are very good at stimulating the liver to create them. Davis says as long as carbohydrate consumption is sustained, the body continuously manufactures triglycerides, resulting in more small LDL particles.

*"Carbohydrates possess the unique capacity
to stimulate insulin, which in turn triggers
fatty acid synthesis in the liver, a process that
floods the bloodstream with triglycerides."*

— Dr. William Davis, *Wheat Belly*

In a study by Dr. Jeff Volek at the University of Connecticut, when participants reduced their carbohydrate intake to 10 percent of total calories over a twelve-week period, small LDL particles were reduced by 26 percent. This study suggests that reducing wheat consumption is an important component of heart health.

Chapter 10: Key Points

- Small LDL particles can cause plaque to form in arteries, which can cause heart disease and strokes.

- When carbohydrates stimulate insulin production, they trigger the synthesis of triglycerides, which in turn contribute to the development of small LDL particles.

- Reducing wheat consumption has been shown to reduce the number of small LDLs, lowering the risk of heart disease and strokes.

IT'S ALL IN YOUR HEAD:
WHEAT AND THE BRAIN

Overview

According to Davis, while scientists are just beginning to understand the effects that wheat consumption has on the brain, there is some evidence that wheat damages brain tissue. Certain types of ataxia (loss of full control of body movements), neuropathy (a disease or dysfunction of the nerves), and encephalopathy (any disease in which some agent affects the functioning of the brain) show some correlation to gluten sensitivity and/or high blood glucose levels. While these conditions are progressive, they may show some improvement when wheat is eliminated from the diet.

> *"Among the most disturbing of wheat's effects are those exerted on brain tissue itself—not 'just' on thoughts and behavior, but on the cerebrum, cerebellum, and other nervous system structures, with consequences ranging from incoordination to incontinence, from seizures to dementia."*
>
> — Dr. William Davis, *Wheat Belly*

Chapter Summary

In Chapter 4, we learned that wheat can bind with morphine receptors on the brain, creating exorphins that affect moods and cravings. In this chapter, Davis explores the effects of wheat on brain tissue. He cites three particular brain disorders that may result from a diet high in wheat.

Cerebellar ataxia causes impaired coordination and balance, and eventually loss of all bodily functions. While the cause is often unknown, Davis notes that 50 percent of those with unexplained ataxia have abnormal blood markers showing gluten sensitivity. The destructive immune response accountable for the gastrointestinal signs of celiac disease can also cause an immune attack on brain cells. The antigliadin antibodies (gliadin is the protein found in gluten; antigliadin antibodies are produced in response to gluten) can bind to cells that are unique to the cerebellum, the part of the brain impaired in ataxia.

Gluten encephalopathy presents as migraines and incoordination, and can lead to dementia and temporal lobe (the part of the brain that organizes sensory input) seizures. Davis reports that 1 percent to 5.5 percent of all celiac sufferers are likely to be diagnosed with these seizures. Studies show that when wheat and gluten are eliminated from the diet, temporal lobe seizures improve.

Peripheral neuropathy affects the nerves in the legs, pelvis, and other organs; high blood sugar levels, sustained over several years, damage the nerves. A common cause is diabetes. Unlike brain cells, peripheral nerve cells can repair themselves to some extent, although not completely. Some studies show eliminating wheat from the diet results in improvement in peripheral neuropathy.

Gluten is the component of wheat most commonly associated with autoimmune phenomena. However, Davis suggests there are other components of wheat that can be equally harmful. Wheat exorphins, for example, can lead to addictive reactions to wheat consumption. And glucose-insulin reactions caused by the high glycemic index of wheat can lead to peripheral neuropathy.

Scientists are just beginning to understand the ways that wheat affects the brain. Diagnoses are complicated by the fact that there is not a consistent set of symptoms but rather a variety of neurological responses. At this point, Davis's best recommendation is to avoid consuming wheat.

"The research into the relationship of wheat, gluten, and brain damage is still preliminary, with many unanswered questions remaining, but what we do know is deeply troubling."

— Dr. William Davis, *Wheat Belly*

Chapter 11: Key Points

- A high incidence of people who suffer from cerebellar ataxia also have abnormal markers for gluten.

- Gluten encephalopathy can cause temporal lobe seizures and dementia; it is triggered by an immune response to wheat.

- Peripheral neuropathy, a condition marked by damage to the peripheral nerves of the legs, pelvis, and other organs, is caused by sustained high blood sugars over several years.

- Wheat's effects on the brain are not fully understood, but preliminary research points to troubling links between wheat and destruction of brain and nerve cells.

BAGEL FACE: WHEAT'S DESTRUCTIVE EFFECT ON THE SKIN

Overview

The skin is the largest organ in the body, and is not immune from the effects of wheat. Wheat can age the skin because it increases the production of AGEs, which cause wrinkles and loss of elasticity. But acne, rashes, and hair loss can also be caused by high blood sugar levels or immune responses associated with wheat or gluten intolerances. Davis suggests that when wheat is eliminated from the diet, these conditions not only improve but also may be reversed.

> *"Wheat expresses itself—actually, the body's reaction to wheat expresses itself—through the skin. . . . Skin changes generally do not occur in isolation: If an abnormality due to wheat is expressed on the skin surface, then it usually means that the skin is not the only organ experiencing an unwanted response."*
>
> — Dr. William Davis, *Wheat Belly*

Chapter Summary

The complexions of contemporary cultures who eat a diet free of wheat and sugar are acne-free. Insulin stimulates the release of the hormone IGF-1 (introduced in Chapter 8), which promotes tissue growth in hair follicles, and, together with insulin itself, stimulates production of sebum, an oily protective film. Skin tissue growth and overproduction of sebum lead to acne.

Dairy is also a culprit, Davis says. It's not the fat content, but the high glycemic index of dairy products like cow's milk, which in turn triggers insulin production. A study of college students found that those who ate the lowest glycemic index diet had a nearly 50 percent reduction in acne.

Dermatitis herpetiformis, or DH, is an itchy, bumpy skin inflammation that reflects an immune response to gluten. DH can manifest as oral ulcers, rashes, bruising, and lesions, and can be treated with strict elimination of wheat and gluten sources. According to Davis, people who suffer from DH do not experience the typical gastrointestinal symptoms of celiac disease but do still show evidence of intestinal inflammation and damage to the small intestine.

After acne, DH is the most common skin response to wheat gluten. But there is a long list of wheat gluten–related skin problems that can be improved or cured by eliminating wheat gluten from the diet.

When wheat provokes an immune response in the skin, hair loss can follow. Alopecia areata is a condition in which hair follicles become inflamed and lose their ability to hold on to individual hairs. Alopecia areata most commonly results in bald patches on the scalp, but, in extreme cases, it can leave a person hairless from head to toe. As with the other skin conditions mentioned in this chapter, Davis suggests that eliminating wheat can reverse this condition.

---

*"[S]kin conditions triggered by wheat gluten range
from simple nuisance to disfiguring disease. . . .
[I]n the aggregate, they add up to an impressive
list of socially disruptive, emotionally difficult,
and physically disfiguring conditions."*

— Dr. William Davis, *Wheat Belly*

Chapter 12: Key Points

- Foods like wheat and dairy that trigger an increase in blood sugar and insulin are the likely cause of acne; removal of wheat should reduce acne.

- Dermatitis herpetiformis, a skin inflammation, reflects an immune response to wheat gluten that can result in rashes, sores, and bruising.

- Wheat consumption can cause hair follicles to become inflamed and unable to hold individual hairs; this condition, known as alopecia areata, often results in bald spots.

13

GOODBYE, WHEAT: CREATE A HEALTHY, DELICIOUS, WHEAT-FREE LIFE

Overview

While a desire to change eating habits seems obvious, making that change can present energy, mood, and willpower challenges. Davis suggests that committing to a wheat-free lifestyle and enduring the necessary wheat withdrawal will be worth it in the end, promising better health, increased weight loss, and improved happiness. Fill the gap left by wheat with vegetables, nuts, meats, eggs, avocados, olives, cheese—in other words, unprocessed, whole foods.

> *"Let me describe a typical person with wheat deficiency: slender, flat tummy, low triglycerides, high HDL ('good') cholesterol, normal blood sugar, normal blood pressure, high energy, good sleep, normal bowel function."*
>
> — Dr. William Davis, *Wheat Belly*

Chapter Summary

As we've learned over the course of *Wheat Belly*, removing wheat from the diet has the potential for incredible health-related benefits. Davis

40

says that because a wheat-free diet improves gastrointestinal health, it also promotes enhanced absorption of vitamin B12, folate, iron, zinc, and magnesium. Without the presence of appetite-stimulating exorphins that wheat creates, hunger and cravings between meals disappear and the body no longer experiences the glucose-insulin cycle every two hours.

The best way to eliminate wheat is all at once—although about 30 percent of people who do so will experience wheat withdrawal, including fatigue, mental fogginess, irritability, low mood, and sadness. These symptoms usually only last a week or two.

It is important to note that simply removing wheat will not eliminate all health issues. Many modern, processed foods affect the body's blood glucose levels in much the same way that wheat does. Davis recommends strictly controlling carbohydrate consumption and avoiding all processed foods. He includes a recommended diet following these guidelines:

- Eat vegetables: Vegetables are rich in nutrients and should make up the majority of the diet.
- Eat *some* fruit: Fruits are high in sugars and should be consumed in limited quantities.
- Eat raw nuts: Nuts are filling and full of fiber, monounsaturated fats, and protein.
- Use oils generously: Stick with healthy oils like extra-virgin olive oil, coconut oil, avocado oil, and cocoa butter, but avoid frying, which triggers AGE formation in oil.
- Eat meats and eggs: Try to eat meat from grass-fed livestock.
- Eat dairy products: Full-fat cheeses can be enjoyed without limit, while other dairy sources should be limited to one to two servings per day.

- Odds and ends: Olives, avocados, pickled vegetables, and raw seeds provide variety. Flaxseed is the one grain that is free of carbohydrates that increase blood sugar; it can be eaten freely.

"If the gap left by wheat is filled with vegetables, nuts, meats, eggs, avocados, olive, cheese—i.e. real food—then not only won't you develop a dietary deficiency, you will enjoy better health, more energy, better sleep, weight loss, and reversal of all the abnormal phenomena we've discussed."

— Dr. William Davis, *Wheat Belly*

Chapter 13: Key Points

- Removing wheat from the diet improves nutrient absorption, reduces calorie consumption, and eliminates the desperate need to replenish the body's glucose levels every two hours.

- Wheat withdrawal can cause fatigue, mental fogginess, and irritability, although these signs typically fade after about a week.

- To be truly healthy, wheat elimination is not enough; a healthy diet contains no wheat or processed foods, and strictly limits carbohydrates.

CONCLUSION

Wheat makes up the largest part of Americans' diets—more than any other food group or type. A look at your average grocery store reveals aisles dominated by wheat breads, wheat cereals, wheat snacks, wheat pastas, and even wheat frozen dinners. Combine this wheat overload with national health guidelines that stress the importance of a diet high in whole grains, and you get a nation of people who suffer from wheat belly. According to Davis, incidences of diabetes and prediabetes, heart disease, and celiac disease—all conditions linked to wheat consumption—are on the rise. Wheat affects weight, complexion, sleep, mood, and immunity, and yet Americans continue to consume it in unprecedented amounts.

Wheat Belly explores the rewards of a life without wheat. Davis asserts that eliminating wheat lowers blood sugar, AGE, triglyceride, and small LDL particle levels, decreases insulin and visceral fat production, and leads to rapid and dramatic weight loss. Removing wheat also improves bone and joint health, heart health, and brain health. According to Davis, a life without wheat is a longer, healthier, and happier life.

CPSIA information can be obtained at www.ICGtesting.com
Printed in the USA
LVOW051836070213

319145LV00001B/255/P